SEXUAL ADDICTION

THE WAY OUT
OF THE WEB

BY JUNE HUNT

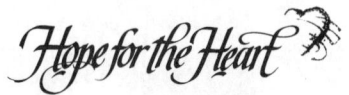

P.O. Box 7 • Dallas, Texas • 75221

Scripture taken from the HOLY BIBLE, NEW INTERNATIONAL VERSION. NIV. Copyright 1973, 1978, 1984 by International Bible Society. Used by permission of Zondervan Publishing House.
All rights reserved.

ISBN: 0-9711792-3-9

To order the Heart of the Matter Series on Sexual Addiction
or other material and tapes related to this topic,
write HOPE FOR THE HEART • P.O. Box 7 • Dallas, TX • 75221
or call toll-free **1-800-488-HOPE (4673).**
www.hopefortheheart.org

Dear friend,

Never will I forget the week I took my mother to visit her dear friend Susan. We arrived around midnight, and the next morning we visited her well-attended, warm-spirited church.

As the service began, I became aware that the media was present, but the pastor was not. I later learned that the young pastor, a gifted Bible teacher, had been arrested for soliciting a prostitute.

Later that day, I made the comment to Susan, "What's so sad is that his wife is going to be blamed for not *meeting his needs*." Stunned, Susan confided, "Why, that's exactly what I was thinking! I had just assumed that if she had met his needs, he wouldn't have gone to a prostitute."

Very simply, I explained, "No one can make another person engage a prostitute or commit any sin. She can't make her husband sin—she doesn't have that power! That was his *choice*. Basically, he has inner needs that are not being met, and he is trying to satisfy them illegitimately." The truth is, this couple's sexual relationship may be normal. Yet, as is the case with many married men who give in to temptation, he was seeking illicit sexual relations rather than bonding with his wife.

Most likely, his wife experienced intense confusion—knowing that they weren't actually sharing true intimacy. In reality, his sexual relationship was not with his wife, but rather with sexual passion.

As God would have it, I had just finished writing much of the material found in this book, and by the end of that same day, the pastor had in his hands a copy of our *Counseling Keys* on Sexual Addiction. The very next day he called to request a copy for each of the elders, hoping they too would gain understanding and insight.

Too many people—men, women and teenagers in epidemic proportions—are shackled to the shame of sexual addiction. And a large percentage feel they are caught in a web and are too entrapped to get out.

But for those who are trapped within the sinister net of this web, there is hope. Matthew 19:26 says that *"with God all things are possible."* The Lord can deliver anyone from the web of sexual addiction. I pray that, by the power of God's word and the practical principles contained within these pages, you or some-one you know will experience the way out and live in true freedom.

Yours in the Lord's hope,

June

SEXUAL ADDICTION
THE WAY OUT OF THE WEB

Sexual Addiction
The Way Out of the Web

"A leopard can't change its spots." This old cliché is true of leopards, but is it also true of people? Particularly those with sexually spotted lives? Many a man has been told, "You'll never change." Many women hear, "You are a bad seed." Do you think it's *impossible* for people to change . . . or perhaps that *you* can't change? The Bible says, *"With God all things are possible"* (Matthew 19:26). Even if you feel that your mind and your heart are defiled, remember God is a Redeemer—He is your Deliverer!

"You, O LORD, have delivered my soul
from death, my eyes from tears,
my feet from stumbling,
that I may walk before the LORD
in the land of the living."
(Psalm 116:8-9)

DEFINITIONS

What is the Scope of Sexual Addiction?

- Sexual addiction is a compulsive, enslaving dependence on erotic excitement resulting in detrimental patterns of thinking and behavior.

- Sexual addiction is immoral. The Greek noun *porneia,* translated in many verses as "fornication" or "immorality," is an umbrella word that covers all forms of sexual immorality.

> *"Put to death, therefore,*
> *whatever belongs to your earthly nature:*
> *sexual immorality, impurity, lust,*
> *evil desires and greed, which is idolatry."*
> *(Colossians 3:5)*

- Sexual addiction is enslaving. The Greek word *douloo* means "to bring under bondage or enslave."

> *"A man is a slave*
> *to whatever has mastered him."*
> *(2 Peter 2:19)*

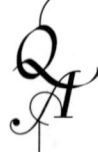

"CAN THOSE WHO HAVE BEEN CAUGHT IN THE SNARE OF SEXUAL ADDICTION BE SET FREE?"

Yes! God's Word gives absolute assurance that anyone can be set free.

"My eyes are ever on the LORD, for only He will release my feet from the snare."
(Psalm 25:15)

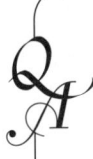

"PORNOGRAPHY IS HARMLESS, SO WHY SHOULD IT BE ILLEGAL?"

- Pornography is addictive and often leads to abuse of others.

- The National Center for Missing and Exploited Children investigated 1,400 cases of child sexual exploitation. Upon arrest, all prosecuted adults were found with various forms of pornography—in most cases child porn.

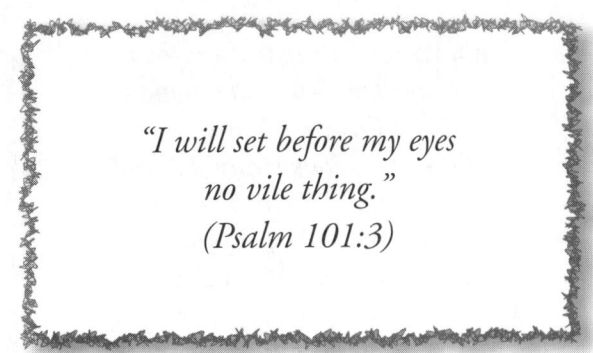

*"I will set before my eyes
no vile thing."
(Psalm 101:3)*

What are the Streets into Sexual Addiction?

- Advertisements—*lingerie, perfume, catalogs*

- Adult book stores, bars and night clubs

- Cards—*postcards, playing cards, photographs*

- Computers—*Internet sites, sex chat rooms and games*

- Movies—*slasher films, X-rated*

- Music—*sexually explicit lyrics*

- Nude beaches and nudist camps

- Peep show booths and massage parlors

- Pornographic literature—*books, magazines, cartoons, comics*

- Telephone—*dial-a-porn 900-numbers, phone sex*

- Television—*cable, soap operas, videos*

"Above all else, guard your heart,
for it is the wellspring of life.
Put away perversity. . . .
Let your eyes look straight ahead,
fix your gaze directly before you.
Make level paths for your feet
and take only ways that are firm.
Do not swerve to the right or the left;
keep your foot from evil."
(Proverbs 4:23-27)

What is the Springboard into Sexual Quicksand?

For **most** people who are sinking in the sands of sexual addiction, their first introduction to pornography came during childhood. The idyllic picture of innocent children building castles in the sand is too often marred by the quicksand of sexual abuse.

PORNOGRAPHY

Pornography is the depiction of erotic behavior intended to arouse sexual, lustful excitement.

- The word *pornography* is from the Greek word *pornē,* which means "harlot."

- *Pornography* debases sexuality and ridicules Christian values in favor of lust and immorality.

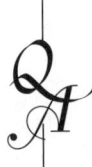

"SINCE GOD CREATED THE HUMAN BODY AS SEXUAL, WHAT'S WRONG WITH NUDITY AND PORNOGRAPHY?"

God created the sexual body for intimacy in marriage and for procreation. On the contrary, pornography is designed simply to arouse indiscriminate sexual lust.

"You have heard that it was said, 'Do not commit adultery.' But I tell you that anyone who looks at a woman lustfully has already committed adultery with her in his heart." (Matthew 5:27-28)

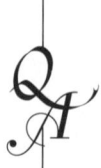

"SINCE PORNOGRAPHY AROUSES SEXUAL DESIRES, WON'T IT ENHANCE OUR SEX LIFE?"

Pornography will hinder your marriage and home life.

Pornography typically leads to:

— *devaluation of the mate*. Love turns to lust for the "ideal" woman portrayed.

— *forced perversion onto the mate*. Men often try to get wives to participate in the perverted acts they have seen.

— *adultery*. Pornography encourages indiscriminate sex.

— *children becoming addicted*. They are often used and abused.

"'You will bear the consequences of your lewdness and your detestable practices,' declares the LORD." (Ezekiel 16:58)

SOFT-CORE PORN

- *Soft-core* porn is the depiction of adult nudity or non-explicit sexual activity between adults.

- *Soft-core* porn is usually not illegal.

- Some examples are: *Playboy, Hustler, Penthouse, Playgirl.*

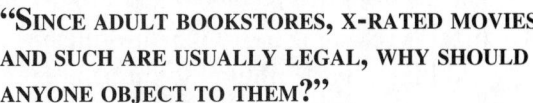

"SINCE ADULT BOOKSTORES, X-RATED MOVIES AND SUCH ARE USUALLY LEGAL, WHY SHOULD ANYONE OBJECT TO THEM?"

Just because something is legal doesn't make it morally right. Lawmakers often respond to pressures of lobbyists or the most vocal special interest groups, settling for less than the excellence set by God's moral law.

"Do not follow the crowd in doing wrong. When you give testimony in a lawsuit, do not pervert justice by siding with the crowd."
(Exodus 23:2)

"ARE ALL SEXUALLY EXPLICIT MATERIALS PORNOGRAPHIC?"

No. A scientific presentation designed to teach or inform would not be considered pornographic. A presentation of the human body from an artist's viewpoint may not necessarily be considered pornographic.

"A discerning man keeps wisdom in view, but a fool's eyes wander to the ends of the earth."
(Proverbs 17:24)

HARD-CORE PORN

- *Hard-core porn* is the depiction of explicit or bizarre sexual activity which is clearly offensive and blatantly degrading to human beings.

- *Hard-core porn* is the street term for "obscene," which means it is illegal.

- *Hard-core porn* can include urinating, defecating or vomiting on another.

Pornographic Material

Heterosexual porn depicts explicit sex acts between males and females, including oral and group sex.

God's Mandate

"Marriage should be honored by all, and the marriage bed kept pure, for God will judge the adulterer and all the sexually immoral." *(Hebrews 13:4)*

Pornographic Material

Homosexual porn depicts explicit sex acts between members of the same sex.

God's Mandate

"Do not lie with a man as one lies with a woman; that is detestable." (Leviticus 18:22)

Pornographic Material

Kiddie porn depicts children having sex with adults and with other children. Child porn is illegal to own or produce and is especially used by pedophiles. (Pedophilia is a sexual perversion in which children are the preferred sexual objects.)

God's Mandate

"If anyone causes one of these little ones who believe in Me to sin, it would be better for him to be thrown into the sea with a large millstone tied around his neck." (Mark 9:42)

Pornographic Material

Bestiality porn depicts sexual activity with animals such as dogs, horses, pigs or donkeys.

God's Mandate

"Cursed is the man who has sexual relations with any animal." (Deuteronomy 27:21)

Pornographic Material

Sexual devices porn depicts the use of "toys" such as mousetraps, fishhooks and rings on the sexual anatomy. In bondage sex, other devices such as handcuffs, wristcuffs, ankle cuffs, bedpost straps, passion paddles and chains are used to depict dominance and submission.

God's Mandate

We should line up with King David's conviction— *"Men of perverse heart shall be far from me; I will have nothing to do with evil." (Psalm 101:4)*

Pornographic Material

Sadomasochistic porn depicts torture of all kinds, including bondage, rape, mutilation and murder. Slasher films and snuff films are X-rated movies containing perverted sex acts and extreme violence culminating in murder.

God's Mandate

"Don't you know that you yourselves are God's temple and that God's Spirit lives in you? If anyone destroys God's temple, God will destroy him; for God's temple is sacred, and you are that temple." (1 Corinthians 3:16-17)

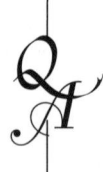

"WHAT DETERMINES IF MATERIAL IS CLASSIFIED AS ILLEGAL?"

Material classified as illegal varies from country to country. However, in most countries, that which is obscene is considered illegal. For example, in the 1973 case of *Miller v. California*, the U.S. Supreme Court established a three-part test to define what is legally obscene.

Pornography which is obscene

— appeals to lustful interests

— depicts clearly offensive sexual conduct

— lacks serious literary, realistic, political or scientific value

Obscenity appeals to, and even urges, vileness instead of virtue. Obscenity degrades the value of human life.

"Among you there must not be even a hint of sexual immorality, or of any kind of impurity, or of greed, because these are improper for God's holy people. Nor should there be obscenity, foolish talk or coarse joking, which are out of place."
(Ephesians 5:3-4)

"SINCE WE CAN'T LEGISLATE MORALITY, WHY IS THERE SO MUCH CONCERN ABOUT PORNOGRAPHY?"

We can legislate morality, and we do. Most laws deal with morality—many Biblical laws such as those against murder, lying and stealing are seen in the laws of every civilized society.

Biblical Example: See the Ten Commandments, Exodus 20:3-17.

CHARACTERISTICS

The Symptoms of Sexual Addiction

Not everyone who is sexually immoral is sexually addicted. While all adulterers and rapists are sex offenders, such offenders are not all sex addicts. (Rape is a power play emanating from anger.) What constitutes a sexual addiction? Within the heart of every addict is a sense of shame—shame because of feeling unlovable, unworthy and unwanted, shame resulting from repeated failure. This shame within an addict produces behavior and beliefs that are most predictable.

*"When wickedness comes,
so does contempt,
and with shame
comes disgrace."
(Proverbs 18:3)*

WHAT CONSTITUTES
A SEXUAL ADDICTION?

Is your sexual activity . . .

SECRETIVE—   not within normal cultural boundaries?
(living a double life)

HOLLOW—   not a relationship with a spouse, but a
relationship with sexual passion?
(prioritizing sexual passion over people)

ABUSIVE—   not uplifting to yourself or others, but
degrading to both?
(exploiting others and debasing yourself)

MOOD-ALTERING— not facing difficult feelings, but seeking
an emotional quick fix?
*(using sexual passion for comfort or to
avoid working through the pain)*

ESSENTIAL—   not indicative that you can live without sexual passion?
*(convincing yourself that sex is the most
important thing in life)*

*"For a man is a slave to
whatever has mastered him."*
(2 Peter 2:19)

The Spiral of Sexual Addiction

The dual world of Jekyll and Hyde is strangely similar to the real and fantasy worlds of the sex addict. Dr. Jekyll's curiosity prompted him to experiment on himself. Yet, to his horror, the harrowing Mr. Hyde increasingly took over his very person. As he retreated from significant relationships for fear of exposure, his thinking became skewed, even to the extreme of losing touch with reality. In the end, for the betterment of society, it seemed Jekyll's only solution was . . . kill Hyde!

Curiosity: A seemingly harmless temptation to look at sexual objects.

> *"Each one is tempted when, by his own evil desire, he is dragged away and enticed."*
> *(James 1:14)*

Addiction: A recurring stimulus in the brain. When a person experiences significant stimulation, the hormone epinephrine is secreted into the blood stream by the adrenal gland. Epinephrine stamps emotional memories into the brain. These memories continue to surface regardless of the person's desire to forget.

> *"Do not be deceived: God cannot be mocked. A man reaps what he sows." (Galatians 6:7)*

Compulsive Masturbation: A response of sexual self-comfort to relieve the arousal. This act becomes part of a sexual ritual.

> *"I will not be mastered by anything."*
> *(1 Corinthians 6:12)*

Escalation: The need for more shocking and explicit sexuality to be stimulated.

> *"Having lost all sensitivity, they have given themselves over to sensuality so as to indulge in every kind of impurity, with a continual lust for more." (Ephesians 4:19)*

Desensitization: The shocking becomes acceptable and unstimulating.

> *"Are they ashamed of their loathsome conduct? No, they have no shame at all; they do not even know how to blush." (Jeremiah 6:15)*

Acting Out: A compulsion to act out what has been seen and imagined because the visual experience is no longer satisfying in itself.

> *"The acts of the sinful nature are obvious: sexual immorality, impurity and debauchery." (Galatians 5:19)*

Despair: Utter disgust over the behavior and total hopelessness to change.

> *"I do not understand what I do. For what I want to do I do not do, but what I hate I do." (Romans 7:15)*

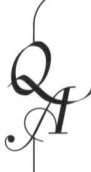

"ARE THERE SOME ADDICTIONS PEOPLE CAN NEVER OVERCOME?"

No, addicts can be rescued from any addiction.

"What I do is not the good I want to do; no, the evil I do not want to do—this I keep on doing. . . . What a wretched man I am! Who will rescue me from this body of death? Thanks be to God—through Jesus Christ our Lord!" (Romans 7:19, 24-25)

*"No temptation has seized you
except what is common to man.
And God is faithful; He will not let you
be tempted beyond what you can bear.
But when you are tempted,
He will also provide a way out
so that you can stand up under it."
(1 Corinthians 10:13)*

The Stages of Sexual Addiction

He grew up in a seemingly normal home—no physical or sexual abuse, yet all his victims were sexually abused, and even mutilated. Eventually he confessed to the murders of 23 young women. How did this man regress from Boy Scout troop to death row? The day before Ted Bundy was executed, he said, "I've met a lot of men motivated to commit violence just like me. And without exception, every one of them was consumed by an addiction to pornography." Just as pornography is progressive, all sexual addiction, if not stopped, progresses into more blatant and risky behavior. What was once sexually stimulating becomes ineffective. More explicit acts are required to create the same sensual excitement.

Stages of Sexual Addiction

Stage 1

Activities

Pornography
Masturbation
Promiscuity
Homosexuality
Prostitution
Cross-dressing
Fetishism
Sex talk lines/chat rooms

Consequences

Low risk
Some behavior illegal
Occasional job threat
Usually considered victimless

Stage 2

Activities

Obscene phone calls
Voyeurism (watching others, being a Peeping Tom)
Exhibitionism
Sexual Harassment

Consequences

Moderate risk
Always illegal
Possible job loss
Always involves a victim

Stage 3

Activities

Child Molestation

Pedophilia

Incest

Rape

Sadomasochistic sex

Consequences

High risk

Always illegal

Probable job loss

Always involves a victim

* This chart is adapted from material in *Out of the Shadows,* by Patrick Carnes, pp. 54-55.

***Do not be deceived.
Activities thought harmless
by the world's standards can be
deadly to the body, soul and spirit.***

*"Do not deceive yourselves. If any one of you thinks
he is wise by the standards of this age, he should
become a 'fool' so that he may become wise.
For the wisdom of this world
is foolishness in God's sight."
(1 Corinthians 3:18-19)*

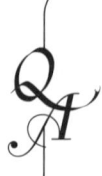

"At what point does the normal sexual desire turn into lust?"

Evaluate what is natural and what is unnatural. It is natural to be attracted to someone, but it is unnatural to sexualize a person. The battle begins in the mind, where uncontrolled thoughts are allowed to move into lustful desires.

"Anyone who looks at a woman lustfully has already committed adultery with her in his heart." (Matthew 5:28)

The Cycle of Sexual Addiction

The Setup

No one lives with more shame, isolation and fear of alienation than the sex addict. Addicts feel they can't help the way they are. Each time they surrender to sexual temptation, sin's tenacious grip gets a stronger hold on their hearts. Sexual addicts believe that the only solution to get their love needs met is through sexual stimulation. Their minds and bodies are held captive to sexual passion.

"For what I do is not the good I want to do; no, the evil I do not want to do—this I keep on doing. Now if I do what I do not want to do, it is no longer I who do it, but it is sin living in me that does it." (Romans 7:19-20)

Worthless Feelings

- "I can't control my sexual urges."

- "I feel like a failure."

- "I'm not a good person."

Withdrawal

- "I can't trust people."

- "If they knew what I've done, they would be disgusted."

- "If they knew the real me, they would reject me."

Wrong Assumptions

- "Sex is my greatest need in life."

- "Sex is the solution to my need for love."

- "Sex is the solace for all my pain."

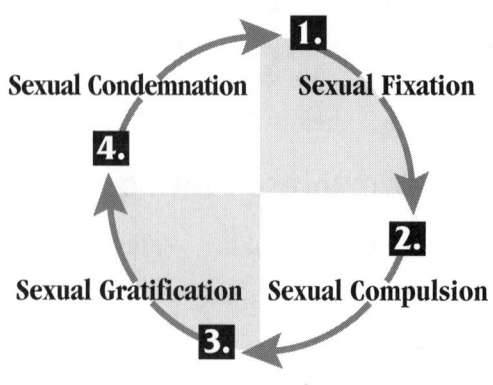

Sexual Condemnation

Sexual Fixation

4.

1.

Sexual Gratification

Sexual Compulsion

3.

2.

The Sequence

*"After desire has conceived, it gives birth to sin;
and sin, when it is full-grown, gives birth to death."*
(James 1:15)

1. Sexual Fixation

An erotic, trance-like state in which obsessing on sex becomes a sedative for the addict's emotional pain.

2. Sexual Compulsion

Compulsive ritualistic routines heighten the excitement and intensify the addict's sexual arousal (cruising, pornography, stalking).

3. Sexual Gratification

Feeling a total loss of self-control, the addict commits the actual sex act.

4. Self Condemnation

Following on the heels of this intoxicating sexual experience comes shame, condemnation and hopelessness. Left with self-contempt and self-loathing, the addict looks for relief, and the sexual cycle perpetuates itself by escaping into the mood-altering fixation on sex.

"The one who sows to please his sinful nature,
from that nature will reap destruction;
the one who sows to please the Spirit,
from the Spirit will reap eternal life."
(Galatians 6:8)

The Solution

The last thing sexual addicts need is rejection, although rejection is usually the first thing that occurs when they are found out. Addicts who live emotionally isolated because of their fear of discovery need emotional connection, heart-to-heart sharing, friend-to-friend commitment. Because sexual addiction is an obsessive relationship with erotic passion, healing comes through secure relationships with caring people. A safe place for addicts to begin opening up and moving out of their secret cesspools is an accountability group of fellow strugglers or friends—ultimately people who can "hate the sin, but truly love the sinner."

"There is a friend
who sticks closer than a brother."
(Proverbs 18:24)

CAUSES

The Birth of an Addiction

YOUR BELIEFS

We've all asked ourselves, "Why did I do that?" The answer is simple: our beliefs birth our behaviors. The messages we received in childhood, especially regarding our own worth, relationships and sexuality, formed our beliefs. These beliefs are powerful, for from them come all our priorities, choices, habits and, yes, even our addictions.

BASIC BELIEFS

Everyone has three inner needs for love, for significance and for security. If—in childhood—these God-given needs were not met, your beliefs reflected that painful lack of nurturing, and you attempted to fill the void. The sex addict believes that sexual passion is comforting and nurturing and that a sexual experience will meet those needs. Since people are undependable, the addict does not risk a relationship with a person, but enters into a relationship with passion. People and things are merely the stimuli used. Since the desire of those who are addicted is passion, their relationship is with passion.

The Need for Love

Basic Belief: "I am unlovable."

"If you really knew me, you wouldn't love me."

"I am bad—bad things should happen to me."

— feeling that no one really cares

— feeling that people care only if they can get something

Result: "I must be *in control* to protect myself."

Enters into a "relationship with sex" not based on love

Example: A relationship with passion,
but using a wife

A relationship with passion,
but using a prostitute

A relationship with passion,
but using a child

The Need for Significance

Basic belief: "I am unworthy."

"If you really knew me, you wouldn't value me."

"I have failed—I'm a failure."

— feeling insignificant

— feeling at fault for everything

Result: "I must be *in charge* to protect myself."

Enters into a "relationship with sex" which can't threaten the addict's significance

Example: A relationship with passion by being a Peeping Tom

A relationship with passion by being a flasher

A relationship with passion by being a rapist

The Need for Security

Basic belief: "I am unwanted."

"If you really knew me, you would abandon me."

"I've lost hope in people—I'm hopeless."

— can't depend on others to meet my needs

— can't risk rejection

Result: "I must be *self-sufficient* to protect my-self."

Enters into a "relationship with sex" so that security won't be threatened

Example: A relationship with passion by gazing at pornography

A relationship with passion by staring at a stripper

A relationship with passion by watching a peep show

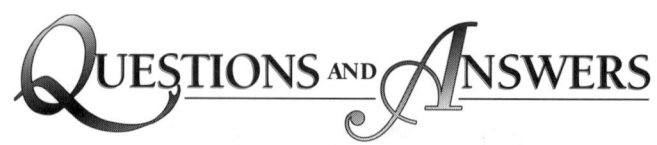

QUESTIONS AND ANSWERS

QUESTION: "CAN MY BELIEFS FROM CHILDHOOD BE CHANGED?"

ANSWER: Yes, you can change your thinking to line up with the Lord's thinking. When your beliefs change, your behavior changes.

"When I was a child, I talked like a child, I thought like a child, I reasoned like a child. When I became a man, I put childish ways behind me." (1 Corinthians 13:11)

QUESTION: "HOW CAN I STOP CALLING SEX TALK LINES WHICH GIVE ME AN INCREDIBLE HIGH? DAY AFTER DAY, MY MIND FEELS INTOXICATED WITH SEX. WHY DO I HAVE THIS CONSTANT CRAVING?"

ANSWER: Although everybody has a God-given need to feel significant, phone sex with a stranger gives a false sense of significance. To be set free of this sexual addiction, replace the false lust for the truth. The truth is that you are so significant that Jesus not only died on the cross for you, but also designed a wonderful plan for your life. Recognize that phone sex will never give you lasting significance. Instead, your significance comes by realizing you were created in the image of God. And you will feel no greater sense of significance than when you are being conformed to the character of Christ.

"Those whom God foreknew He predestined to be conformed to the likeness of His Son." (Romans 8:29)

QUESTION: "HOW CAN I STOP MENTALLY UNDRESSING EVERY ATTRACTIVE WOMAN I SEE?"

ANSWER: The moment you find yourself in the midst of sexual temptation, you must immediately turn:

- Turn your eyes away without delay. Say in your heart, "I refuse to let my eyes lead me into the sexual temptation."

- Turn your mind toward integrity. Declare out loud, "I'm determined to be a man of highest moral integrity."

- Turn in prayer to God. "Lord Jesus, I'm committing myself to be pure in both my mind and my body."

"Everyone who confesses the name of the Lord must turn away from wickedness."
(2 Timothy 2:19)

QUESTION: "HOW CAN I CONTROL MY LUSTFUL FANTASIES? I SIMPLY CAN'T STOP FANTASIZING."

ANSWER: God would never tell you to stop lusting without giving you the power to stop. The starting point for victory is realizing that when a sexual thought flashes into your mind, you must redirect that thought or replace it. Years ago, Martin Luther painted a graphic picture with words to this effect, "You can't keep the birds from flying over your head, but you can keep them from making a nest in your hair." You are the only one who controls how long you will entertain a thought—how long you will dwell on it. Make a commitment—a covenant with your eyes—that you will not maintain a gaze which leads to an immoral thought. And make a covenant with your mind that you will not allow an immoral thought to reside in your heart.

"I made a covenant with my eyes not to look lustfully at a girl." (Job 31:1)

QUESTION: "I AM NOT MARRIED, AND I STRUGGLE WITH MASTURBATION, A HABIT I DEVELOPED AS A TEENAGER. I AM A CHRISTIAN AND THE GUILT IS OVERWHELMING. HOW CAN I OVERCOME THIS SEXUAL ADDICTION?"

ANSWER: Masturbation is not mentioned in Scripture, but a Biblical principle is applicable here.

"'Everything is permissible for me'—but not everything is beneficial. 'Everything is permissible for me'—but I will not be mastered by anything." (1 Corinthians 6:12)

The implication is that anything that has mastery over us is sin because Christ is to be our Master. A major step in gaining mastery over guilt-producing sexual habits is to take immediate control of your thoughts at the first urge.

- Pray that God's highest purpose for your life would be realized "Lord, I'll do whatever it takes to be conformed to Your character."

- Claim the Scripture, *"I can do everything through Him who gives me strength"* (Philippians 4:13).

- Say to yourself, "I have no right to do this to my body. I belong to God. My body is His temple, and I will not defile it! I resist this temptation in Jesus' name."

- Do something positive: sing a hymn, pray a prayer, phone a friend, lend a hand, read the Bible.

As a Christian, you have Christ living in you, imparting to you His divine power to live a godly life.

"His divine power has given us everything we need for life and godliness through our knowledge of Him who called us by His own glory and goodness."
(2 Peter 1:3)

The Double Delusions of Sexual Addiction

Delusions are persistent false beliefs about yourself and others. In other words, "A delusion is believing your own lies." The faulty beliefs of sexual addicts enable them to manufacture and believe their own elaborate defense systems. This interactive process between beliefs and denials results in seriously impaired thinking, moving them further and further from reality.

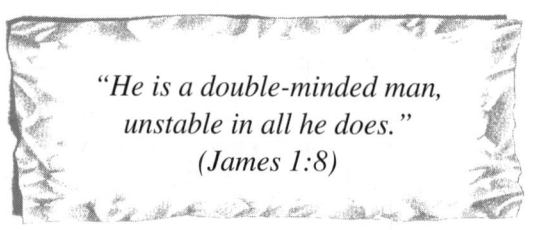

"He is a double-minded man, unstable in all he does."
(James 1:8)

The addict lives in two worlds:
the outward appearance of normalcy
and the inward state of depravity.

Unbridled Beliefs

All people and places, all joys and pains are seen by the addict through a sexual lens.

Distorted Defenses

When behavior is attacked by others or by his own conscience, the addict must employ an army of defenses in an effort not to lose face.

Unbridled Beliefs

Sex is the source of excitement.
Sex is the balm for abuse.

Distorted Defenses

Justifications   "I have to have sex."
"I was molested as a child."

Unbridled Beliefs

Sex is the remedy for rejection.
Sex is the payment for performing well.

Distorted Defenses

Blame Shifting   "You're so unresponsive."
"My boss is too demanding."

Unbridled Beliefs

Sex is the panacea for pain.
Sex is the salve for stress.

Distorted Defenses

Excuses   "I have never felt loved."
"I have to find ways to relax."

Unbridled Beliefs

Sex is the antidote to anger.
Sex is the light for life.

Distorted Defenses

Arguments   "You're out to get me."
"She really did want it and liked it."

Unbridled Beliefs

> Sex is the treatment for tension.
> Sex is the answer to anxiety.

Distorted Defenses

Rationalizations   "I just have to have more sex."
               "I have to relieve the pressure."

Unbridled Beliefs

> Sex is the basis for being.
> Sex is the key to comfort.

Distorted Defenses

Denials   "I didn't do anything wrong."
               "I didn't hurt anyone."

* This chart is adapted from material in *Out of the Shadows,* by Patrick Carnes, Ph.D.

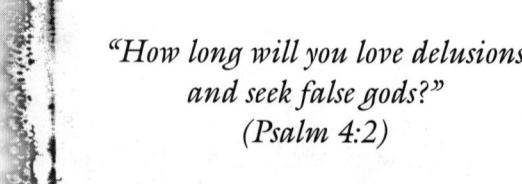

*"How long will you love delusions
and seek false gods?"
(Psalm 4:2)*

The Root Cause
of Sexual Addiction

WRONG BELIEF: "THE MOST IMPORTANT THING IN MY LIFE IS SEX. I WILL DO WHATEVER IS NECESSARY TO GET MY SEXUAL NEEDS MET."

RIGHT BELIEF: "The most important thing in my life is to be changed by an intimate love relationship with Jesus. My first priority is to love my Lord and then to love others with a pure heart. Jesus loved me enough to die for me, and He now lives in me. Because my body belongs to Him, He promises to meet all of my true needs."

"The body is not meant for sexual immorality, but for the Lord, and the Lord for the body. . . . Do you not know that your body is a temple of the Holy Spirit, who is in you, whom you have received from God? You are not your own; you were bought at a price. Therefore honor God with your body."
(1 Corinthians 6:13, 19-20)

STEPS TO SOLUTION

KEY VERSE to Memorize

"Flee from sexual immorality.
All other sins a man commits
are outside his body,
but he who sins sexually
sins against his own body."
(1 Corinthians 6:18)

KEY PASSAGE
to Read and Reread

1 Thessalonians 4:1-8

Whatever God tells you to do, He will equip
you to do. When God calls you to avoid sexual
immorality, you can do it. Don't live as a prisoner
of past defeat. **Claim your high calling**!

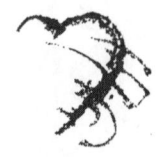

CLAIM YOUR HIGH CALLING

1 Thessalonians 4:1-8

"We instructed you how to live in order to please God, as in fact you are living. Now we ask you and urge you in the Lord Jesus to do this more and more. For you know what instructions we gave you by the authority of the Lord Jesus. It is God's will that you should be sanctified: that you should avoid sexual immorality; that each of you should learn to control his own body in a way that is holy and honorable, not in passionate lust like the heathen, who do not know God; and that in this matter no one should wrong his brother or take advantage of him. The Lord will punish men for all such sins, as we have already told you and warned you. For God did not call us to be impure, but to live a holy life. Therefore, he who rejects this instruction does not reject man but God, who gives you His Holy Spirit."

Why Avoid Immorality?

Because . . .

1 Thessalonians 4

- *You will* please God. *verse 1*

- *You will* prove that you can take instruction from God. *verse 1*

- *You will* respond to the authority of God. *verse 2*

- *You will* be in the will of God. *verse 3*

- *You will* be sanctified (set apart). *verse 3*

- *You will* control your own body. *verse 4*

- *You will* do what is honorable and holy. *verse 4*

- *You will* not display passionate lust. *verse 5*

- *You will* not be like the heathen. *verse 5*

- *You will* not wrong another person. *verse 6*

- *You will* not take advantage of another. *verse 6*

- *You will* not be impure. *verse 7*

- *You will* live up to your holy calling. *verse 7*

- *You will* not be rejecting God. *verse 8*

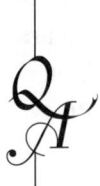

"I RECENTLY BECAME A CHRISTIAN. HOW CAN I CLOSE THE DOOR ON PAST SEXUAL RELATIONSHIPS WITH WOMEN AND MOVE INTO MORALLY PURE RELATIONSHIPS?"

First, admit that each immoral relationship was sinful. Second, ask the Lord to break the bond between you and each woman with whom you have been involved. Then third, present your body as a living sacrifice to the Lord. Last, renew your mind. Whenever you are attracted to a woman, pray, "Lord Jesus, may I see her as You see her through Your eyes. I pray she would grow more and more into the godly woman You created her to be. In Your holy name I pray. Amen."

"Therefore, I urge you, brothers,
in view of God's mercy,
to offer your bodies as living sacrifices,
holy and pleasing to God—
this is your spiritual act of worship.
Do not conform any longer
to the pattern of this world,
but be transformed by the
renewing of your mind.
Then you will be able to test
and approve what God's will is—
His good, pleasing and perfect will."
(Romans 12:1-2)

The Doorway out of Addiction

When you trust Jesus Christ as your Lord and Savior, you are given a new identity. The Bible says you are not just a creation of God, but a child of God. You are *"set apart,"* you are in His family, you receive His nature and are to reflect His character. What an extraordinary privilege! Since sexual sin doesn't reflect Christ, who is in you, you can be assured that He has already provided a way out for you.

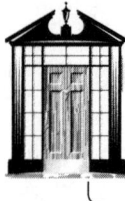

"The One who calls you is faithful and He will do it."
(1 Thessalonians 5:24)

Decide: Do you really want to be set free?

"Am I ready to take responsibility for my addiction?"

"Am I sick and tired of being in this bondage?"

"Am I willing to go to war to win?"

"Prepare your minds for action; be self-controlled." *(1 Peter 1:13)*

Dispel the myth that you don't need help.

"I admit I'm out of control."

"I admit my sexual addiction is sin."

"I admit I can't change myself."

"Create in me a pure heart, O God, and renew a steadfast spirit within me."
(Psalm 51:10)

Deal with the secret of child abuse.

(Some say that over 80 percent of addicts were sexually abused, over 90 percent, emotionally abused.)

Talk with a friend—let go of the secret.

Talk to a counselor in order to understand abuse issues.

Talk to the perpetrator in a safe place—confrontation is Biblical.

"If your brother sins against you, go and show him his fault, just between the two of you. If he listens to you, you have won your brother over. But if he will not listen, take one or two others along." (Matthew 18:15-16)

Discern the inner need you have tried to meet through sexual passion.

Your need for sacrificial love?

Your need for significance?

Your need for security?

"Surely You desire truth in the inner parts; You teach me wisdom in the inmost place." (Psalm 51:6)

Determine to let Jesus meet your needs.

Ask Him to forgive you for your willful sin.

Ask Him to come into your life as your personal Lord and Savior.

Ask Him to meet your deepest inner needs.

"My God will meet all your needs." (Philippians 4:19)

Dedicate your life to the Lord Jesus.

Let His will be your will.

Let the Lord be Lord of your life.

Let Christ have absolute control.

"If anyone would come after Me, he must deny himself and take up his cross daily and follow Me. For whoever wants to save his life will lose it, but whoever loses his life for Me will save it." (Luke 9:23-24)

Prayer of Salvation

*God, I need You in my life.
I admit that my life has been out of control.
Please forgive me for all my sins.
Jesus, thank You for dying on the cross
to pay the penalty for my sin.
I'm asking You to come into my life
to be my Lord and my Savior.
Change me inside out, and make me
the person You want me to be.
In Your holy name I pray. Amen.*

Breaking Free

As bank president, you receive word that a time bomb inside the vault is set to go off at midnight. The combination lock has been electronically jammed. If you don't get rid of the bomb, the bank will be destroyed. You must break the code! Similarly, in every addict's mind a sexual time bomb threatens to destroy both the body and soul. With the right combination you can save yourself if you break the code.

Cracking the Code

The mind of every addict is locked by faulty beliefs. Your beliefs are what you think about your own value, your relationships and your sexuality. They determine all of your behavior. If your thinking is faulty, your findings are faulty, and then the way you function will be faulty.

The Bible says not only that you can change, but also how you can change. Romans 12:2 says, *"Be transformed by the renewing of your mind."* You must reprogram your mind with the right code. Every day for the next twelve weeks read these life-changing truths. Pray that God will open your heart. Jesus says . . . *"The truth will set you free" (John 8:32).*

Your Need for Love

False Belief: **"I am unlovable. . . . Sex gives me the feeling of being loved."**

True Belief: You are loved. . . . God loves you.

- Jesus loved you enough to die on the cross for you.

  "God so loved the world that He gave His one and only Son, that whoever believes in Him shall not perish but have eternal life." (John 3:16)

- Your heavenly Father loved you enough to adopt you into His family.

  "How great is the love the Father has lavished on us, that we should be called children of God! And that is what we are! The reason the world does not know us is that it did not know Him." (1 John 3:1)

Conclusion: Sex is not love, love is not sex—sex is sex. Love is a commitment that seeks the highest and best for another person. Since God loves you in this way, He will give you the ability to develop other loving relationships in which sex is not a substitute for love.

"[Love] is not self-seeking."
(1 Corinthians 13:5)

Your Need for Significance

False belief: **"I am unworthy. . . . Sex makes me feel significant."**

True belief: You already have worth. . . . God has already established your worth.

• God created you. Therefore, you have worth.

"You created my inmost being; You knit me together in my mother's womb." (Psalm 139:13)

• If you are a Christian, you have worth because Christ lives in you.

"To them God has chosen to make known among the Gentiles the glorious riches of this mystery, which is Christ in you, the hope of glory." (Colossians 1:27)

Conclusion: Sex does not give you significance. You are significant because Jesus Himself is in you and imparts His power to you. He is your source of power and significance.

"His divine power has given us everything
we need for life and godliness
through our knowledge of Him
who called us by His own glory
and goodness."
(2 Peter 1:3)

Your Need for Security

False belief: **"I am unwanted. . . . Sex numbs the pain of my insecurity."**

True belief: You are wanted. . . . The Lord wants you.

- The Lord wants to be your Shepherd throughout life.

  "The LORD is my shepherd, I shall not be in want." (Psalm 23:1)

- The Lord wants to walk with you through life.

  "When you pass through the waters, I will be with you; and when you pass through the rivers, they will not sweep over you. When you walk through the fire, you will not be burned; the flames will not set you ablaze." (Isaiah 43:2)

Conclusion: Sex does not give you security. Your security is found in a love relationship with the Lord. This true security can never be taken away from you.

"The Lord Himself goes
before you and will be with you;
He will never leave you nor forsake you.
Do not be afraid; do not be discouraged."
(Deuteronomy 31:8)

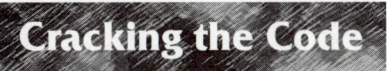

WITH THE FREEDOM FORMULA

Don't Focus
on the Negative Combination

Every time you focus on quitting a sexual obsession, you want it all the more. Living under the "law" never changes you. If you focus only on what you shouldn't do, you will be pulled more powerfully to do it.

- "I need to quit thinking about sex."

- "I won't rent these X-rated movies."

- "I have to get over this addiction."

- "I shouldn't call the sex line."

- "I'll quit cruising next month."

It keeps you focused on what you don't want.

"The power of sin is the law."
(1 Corinthians 15:56)

Focus
on the Positive Combination

A New Purpose

"I want to reflect the character of Christ through what I see and do."

"I am 'predestined to be conformed to the likeness of His Son.'" (Romans 8:29)

+

A New Priority

"I will do whatever it takes to have a pure heart and life."

"Do not conform any longer to the pattern of this world, but be transformed by the renewing of your mind." (Romans 12:2)

+

A New Plan

"I will rely on Christ's strength, not mine."

"I can do everything through Him who gives me strength." (Philippians 4:13)

=

A Transformed Life

God's Gift of Self-Control

To see pornography as sin

To destroy all erotic material

To purchase and read only uplifting material

To avoid tempting situations

To turn quickly to a preplanned project (exercise, hobbies, reading, etc.) when tempted

To think on Philippians 4:8-9 when tempted

To make needed changes in old routines (driving route, television, reading material, etc.)

To block all "adult" X-rated programs from TV, cable, hotels

To resist channel surfing on TV

To be accountable to a friend each week

To memorize and claim pertinent Scriptures

To break the chain of obsession

"Whatever is true, whatever is noble, whatever is right, whatever is pure, whatever is lovely, whatever is admirable— if anything is excellent or praiseworthy— think about such things."
(Philippians 4:8)

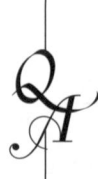

"Although I am Christian, I still have a problem with lust. Now that I know God loves me and has given me eternal life, having these desires makes me feel even worse. Why do I keep wanting to do these things that I know are wrong?"

Paul spoke to this very problem in Romans 7 when he said, *"When I want to do good, evil is right there with me. For in my inner being I delight in God's law; but I see another law at work in the members of my body, waging war against the law of my mind and making me a prisoner of the law of sin at work within my members. What a wretched man I am! Who will rescue me from this body of death?"* Paul goes on to answer his own question by saying the answer is Jesus—relying on the Spirit of Christ who lives in you to be your source of power for change. If you have accepted Christ to be your Lord and Savior, He will give you His divine power to overcome sin.

"You, however, are controlled
not by the sinful nature
but by the Spirit, if the Spirit
of God lives in you."
(Romans 8:9)

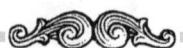

The Pathway to Purity

Does the thought of purity seem impossible to you?
Something unattainable? Take heart. God would
never call you to be pure without giving you all that
you need to be pure. So be encouraged. As you
yield your life to His life, you have God's guaran-
tee that you can have a pure heart and a pure life.

"For God did not call us to be impure,
but to live a holy life."
(1 Thessalonians 4:7)

PURITY

Participate— in an accountability group dealing with
sex addictions.

— Meet regularly and talk specifically
each week.

— Set realistic guidelines and goals.

— Admit each time that you slip.

"Two are better than one, because they
have a good return for their work: If one
falls down, his friend can help him up.
But pity the man who falls and has no one
to help him up!" (Ecclesiastes 4:9-10)

Uphold— boundary lines that must be off limits.

— Write down danger places such as an
addiction room at home.

— Give this information to your accountability partner.

— Lock yourself out of X-rated computer
chat rooms so that you won't know the
code.

"The prudent see danger and take refuge, but the simple keep going and suffer for it." (Proverbs 27:12)

Rid— yourself, your home and work of all sexually addictive items.

— Throw away all pornography.

— Clear away all erotic paraphernalia.

— Discard addresses and calling cards of all sexual contacts.

"Wash and make yourselves clean. Take your evil deeds out of My sight! Stop doing wrong, learn to do right!" (Isaiah 1:16-17)

Incorporate— the power of Christ daily when temptation overwhelms you.

— "Lord, I'm relying on You to be my Redeemer."

— "Lord, I'm depending on You to be my Deliverer."

— "Lord, in my weakness I need Your strength."

" 'My grace is sufficient for you, for My power is made perfect in weakness.' Therefore I will boast all the more gladly about my weaknesses, so that Christ's power may rest on me." (2 Corinthians 12:9)

Take— on positive habits of discipline, such as exercise, sports, regular sleep and new hobbies.

— Choose to make a "to do" list of healthy activities you enjoy.

— Choose to do one item from the list when you are tempted.

— Choose to write a letter, call a friend, or help someone in need.

"He who heeds discipline shows the way to life, but whoever ignores correction leads others astray." (Proverbs 10:17)

Yield— your mind to meditating on and memorizing Scripture.

— Read a chapter from the New Testament each day.

— Read Romans 6 once a week.

— Read *Colossians 3:1-5* each day and memorize *Philippians 4:8-9.*

"Get rid of all moral filth and the evil that is so prevalent and humbly accept the word planted in you, which can save you." (James 1:21)

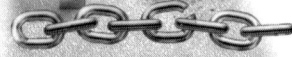

*"No temptation has seized you
except what is common to man.
And God is faithful; He will not
let you be tempted beyond what you
can bear. But when you are tempted,
He will also provide a way out
so that you can stand up under it."
(1 Corinthians 10:13)*

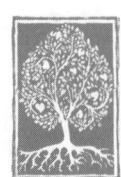

Breaking
Sexual Bonds
and Strongholds

When two people engage in a sexual relationship, a bond is established. Whether the sexual relationship is within marriage or outside of marriage, a bond is still formed. Any sexual relationship outside of one's own marriage needs to be broken, even if it occurred in the past and is over. Begin by praying:

"God, thank You for loving me in spite of my wrong choices. I confess each sexually immoral relationship as sin. Lord Jesus, through Your supernatural power, I ask You to break any unholy sexual bond that exists between me and anyone else. I pray that the bond with ___(names)___ be broken. (Pray this sentence naming each person with whom you have been sexually and/or emotionally involved.) Lord Jesus, from this moment on, I will rely on Your power and live in Your strength."

"Do you not know that he who unites himself
with a prostitute is one with her in body?
For it is said, 'The two will become one flesh.'
But he who unites himself with the Lord
is one with Him in spirit."
(1 Corinthians 6:16-17)

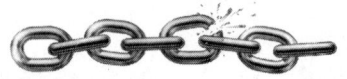

Severing the Stronghold

When a series of sexually impure relationships occur, a sexual stronghold is formed. Until you demolish the stronghold, you will continue in the sexually impure patterns of the past. Pray that the sexual stronghold be demolished.

"Lord Jesus, I affirm that sex is not my master. You are my Master. Through the supernatural power of Christ, I pray that you destroy every stronghold—any mental, emotional or sexual stronghold in my life. Keep me from justifying impure thoughts. May I see sin as you see it and hate sin as you hate it. Lord, I give You control of my life."

"For though we live in the world, we do not wage war as the world does. The weapons we fight with are not the weapons of the world. On the contrary, they have divine power to demolish strongholds. We demolish arguments and every pretension that sets itself up against the knowledge of God, and we take captive every thought to make it obedient to Christ."
(2 Corinthians 10:3-5)

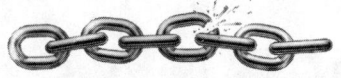

Winning the Spiritual War

The Bible tells us that we are engaged in an ongoing battle—a spiritual war against three enemies; the world, the flesh and the devil.

"As for you, you were dead in your transgressions and sins, in which you used to live when you followed the ways of this world and of the ruler of the kingdom of the air, the spirit who is now at work in those who are disobedient. All of us also lived among them at one time, gratifying the cravings of our sinful nature and following its desires and thoughts. Like the rest, we were by nature objects of wrath." (Ephesians 2:1-3)

— The *word* refers to ideas and lies that are in opposition to God.

"You adulterous people, don't you know that friendship with the world is hatred toward God? Anyone who chooses to be a friend of the world becomes an enemy of God." (James 4:4)

— The *flesh*, sometimes translated "sinful nature," means living out of our own abilities, independently of God.

"I know that nothing good lives in me, that is, in my sinful nature. For I have the desire to do what is good, but I cannot carry it out." (Romans 7:18)

— The *devil*, or *Satan,* is the supreme adversary of God who wants to defeat the followers of God.

"Be self-controlled and alert. Your enemy the devil prowls around like a roaring lion looking for someone to devour." (1 Peter 5:8)

SPIRITUAL WARFARE PRAYER

Whether you realize it or not, you have an enemy of your soul whose purpose is to defeat God's purpose for your life. Although sexual enticement may have been your snare, spiritual warfare can be the means to set you free. Every time you sense the snare of sexual temptation, pray this prayer:

"Heavenly Father, thank You that the blood of Jesus purchased the full forgiveness of my sins and that I am Your child forever. Because Jesus lives in me and because He has supernatural power, I realize that I have His supernatural power to overcome any sin. *(Revelation 12:11) (Colossians 1:27)*

Because Jesus had victory over Satan and his demons, I choose to live in His victory. *(Colossians 2:13-15) (1 Corinthians 15:57)*

In the name of Jesus, I command that any power not from God leave me. No demonic power has authority over me because greater is Jesus who is in me than Satan who is in the world. *(James 4:7) (1 John 4:4)*

Lord God, I ask you to take back any ground the enemy has gained in my mind, will and emotions and to enable me to firmly stand my ground. *(Ephesians 6:13)*

My body is the temple of Your Holy Spirit, and I refuse to allow it to be used for any ungodly purpose. *(1 Corinthians 6:19)*

Put a hedge of protection around my body, a guard around my mind and blinders around my eyes. *(Job 1:10)*

Make me aware of anything that is not pleasing to You. (Psalm 139:23-24)

Conform me to Your character, and fill me with Your Spirit. *(Romans 8:29) (Ephesians 5:18)*

From this moment on, I will rely on Your power and live in Your strength. *(Philippians 4:13)*

In the powerful name of Jesus, I pray. Amen."

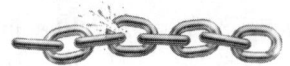

"May God Himself, the God of peace, sanctify you through and through. May your whole spirit, soul and body be kept blameless at the coming of our Lord Jesus Christ. The One who calls you is faithful and He will do it."
(1 Thessalonians 5:23-24)

The Way Out of the Web

Many who have become addicted to pornography on the Internet promise themselves or others they will stop . . . only to keep coming back for more. Even finding ways to get around the Internet filters, blockers, and controls on their computers can become an exciting adventure. Realistically, there are no 100 percent guarantees to keep all addicts from accessing sexually enticing materials, aside from canceling or totally blocking Internet access. However, but there are creative ways to help you get free or regain control. Strategic planning is crucial, and a commitment to the Lord that you want to do whatever He wants you to do will fulfill your promises . . . to yourself and to those who love you.

"You need to persevere
so that when you have done the will of God,
you will receive what He has promised."
(Hebrews 10:36)

- Use a Christian Internet service provider (ISP) which filters the Internet at the server side.

- Use an Internet filter which has a password that must be entered before you can change the controls. (If only your wife possesses the password, she can be your accountability partner. If you are single, choose a trusted friend!)

- If you, like many married men struggle with late-night Internet pornography, use a filter that blocks late-night access. Several Internet guardian programs allow the password holder to limit certain times in which the Internet can be accessed.

- Be sure to find a guardian filter that is guaranteed to work with your Internet browser. (For example, several Christian Internet filters do not block Internet access if someone uses the AOL browser.)

- Find an ISP or an Internet filter that allows the password holder to access a protected file that tracks all Internet activity. This serves as a major reminder that all Internet activity will be monitored. This feature also prohibits the user from erasing history trails.

- Since many people receive pornographic e-mails inviting them to simply click on a link in the e-mail to be immediately transferred to a porn site, be sure that you have a filter that either filters out pornographic e-mail or stops the Internet user from being linked to a pornographic site.

- Place the home computer in a part of the house where there is a lot of traffic and where the computer screen can be easily seen. This can help to avoid the user's being secretive or hidden.

- In many cases, canceling all Internet access for a period of time is necessary to help break the cycle of sexual addiction.

*"Nothing in all creation is hidden from God's sight.
Everything is uncovered and laid bare before
the eyes of Him to whom we must give account."
(Hebrews 4:13)*

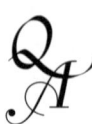

"MY TEENAGE SON IS ADDICTED TO PORNOG-RAPHY—HE REFUSES TO STOP ACCESSING IT ON THE INTERNET. I HAVE REPEATEDLY TOLD HIM TO STOP, BUT TO NO AVAIL. WHAT CAN I DO?"

While an Internet filter should certainly be applied, many network surfers have learned to circumvent the system—nevertheless, you need to communicate your convictions and your boundaries about pornography. You could say:

"Son, I love you and want you to have increased freedom. But I also know pornography has such a strong pull that many people become addicted. That is just one reason why you have been prohibited from accessing porn sites. In reality, pornography poisons your mind while at the same time pollutes our home. Pornography not only violates my values, but also offends the heart of God—because it debases the very human beings whom He made in His image. Since you're having such difficulty with self-control, I see that you need my help. You've left me no choice but to revoke all computer privileges. After a month, we can talk about how you can regain my trust."

Tell him that because you love him, you will do whatever it takes to help him become a young man of moral character. If he has a computer in his room, remove it. No matter how much he says he needs it for school, accessing pornography was his choice; therefore, he has chosen his own consequence.

"If your right eye causes you to sin,
gouge it out and throw it away.
It is better for you to lose one part of your body
than for your whole body to be thrown into hell.
And if your right hand causes you to sin,
cut it off and throw it away."
(Matthew 5:29-30)

Scriptures to Memorize

. . . .

"It is God's will
that you should be sanctified:
*that you should **avoid sexual immorality**."*
(1 Thessalonians 4:3)

"Anyone who looks at a woman lustfully
*has already **committed adultery***
*with her **in his heart**."*
(Matthew 5:28)

*"**Put to death** . . . whatever belongs to*
*your earthly nature: **sexual immorality**,*
impurity, lust, evil desires and greed,
which is idolatry."
(Colossians 3:5)

"Do not be deceived: God cannot
*be mocked. **A man reaps what he sows**.*
*The one who sows to **please** his sinful nature,*
from that nature will reap destruction;
*the one who sows to **please** the Spirit,*
from the Spirit will reap eternal life."
(Galatians 6:7-8)

*"**Do not conform** any longer **to the***
***pattern of this world**, but be transformed*
by the renewing of your mind.
Then you will be able to test
*and approve what **God's will is**—*
His good, pleasing and perfect will."
(Romans 12:2)

*"For God did **not** call us to **be impure**, but to **live a holy life**."*
(1 Thessalonians 4:7)

*"**My eyes** are ever **on the LORD**, for only He will release my feet from the **snare**."*
(Psalm 25:15)

*"I made a **covenant with my eyes not to look lustfully** at a girl."*
(Job 31:1)

*"No temptation has seized you except what is **common to man**. And God is faithful; He will not let you be **tempted beyond what you can bear**. But when you are tempted, He will also provide a way out so that you can stand up under it."*
(1 Corinthians 10:13)

*"**Whatever is true**, whatever is **noble**, whatever is **right**, whatever is **pure**, whatever is **lovely**, whatever is **admirable**— if anything is **excellent** or **praiseworthy**— **think about** such things."*
(Philippians 4:8)

Selected Bibliography

• •

Anderson, Kerby. *Living Ethically in the '90s*. Wheaton, Ill.: Victor, 1990.

Arterburn, Stephen, and Fred Stoeker, with Mike Yorkey. *Every Man's Battle*. Colorado Springs, Colo.: Waterbrook, 2000.

Carnes, Patrick J. *Out of the Shadows: Understanding Sexual Addiction*. Minneapolis, Minn.: CompCare, 1983. [Secular, but authoritative]

Court, J. H., "Pornography." In *Baker Encyclopedia of Psychology*. ed. David G.Benner. Grand Rapids: Baker, 1985.

Daniels, Robert. *The War Within*. Wheaton, Ill.: Crossway, 1997.

Focus on the Family. *Pornography: Addictive, Progressive and Deadly*, Pomona, Calif.: Focus on the Family, 1989. Videocassette.

Focus on the Family. *The Power of the Picture*. Pomona, Calif.: Focus on the Family, 1989.

Focus on the Family. *The Winnable War*. Pomona, Calif.: Focus on the Family, 1989.

Focus on the Family. *The Winnable War*. Pomona, Calif.: Focus on the Family, 1989. Videocassette.

Hall, Laurie. *An Affair of the Mind: One Woman's Courageous Battle to Salvage Her Family from the Devastation of Pornography*. Colorado Springs, Colo.: Focus on the Family, 1996. [Recommended]

Hall, Laurie. *The Cleavers Don't Live Here Anymore*. Ann Arbor, Mich.: Servant, 2000. [Recommended]

Kirk, Jerry. *The Mind Polluters*. Nashville: Thomas Nelson, 1985.

Lutzer, Erwin. *Twelve Myths That Americans Believe*. Chicago: Moody, 1993.

National Coalition for the Protection of Children and their Families. *Sex Addiction: Too Much of a Good Thing.* Cincinnati, Ohio: National Coalition for the Protection of Children and their Families, 1983. [Available at http://www.nationalcoalition.org. June 27,2001]

Olson, Jeff. *When a Man's Eye Wanders: Breaking the Power of Pornography*. Grand Rapids: Radio Bible Class Ministries, 1999.

Perkins, Bill. *When Good Men are Tempted*. Grand Rapids: Zondervan, 1996.

Rogers, Henry J., and Norm Miller. *The Silent War: Ministering to Those Trapped in the Deception of Pornography*. Green Forest, Ark.: New Leaf, 2000. [Recommended]

Schaumberg, Harry. *False Intimacy*. Colorado Springs: NavPress, 1992. [Recommended]

Vine, W. E., Merrill F. Unger, and William White, Jr., eds. *Vine's Expository Dictionary of Biblical Words*. Nashville: Thomas Nelson, 1984.

"The War Within Continues. An Update on a Christian Leader's Struggle with Lust." *Leadership*. (winter 1988): 24-33.

"The War Within: An Anatomy of Lust." *Leadership*. (fall 1982): 30-48.

ℬiblical 𝒞ounseling 𝒦eys . . .

are "people helper" resources based on the fundamental truths of the Bible. Biblical *Keys* are available on approximately 100 topics.

Many of the topics complement or will "come alongside" to help you develop more insight on the subject of *Sexual Addiction*.

RELATED TOPICS

Alcohol & Drug Abuse

Anger

Anxiety

Childhood Sexual Abuse

Codependency

Habits

Rejection

Self-Worth

Stress

Workaholism

For a complete listing of topics,
and to request a product catalog—
call toll free—

1-800-488-HOPE (4673)
www.hopefortheheart.org